The Keto Handbook of Weight Loss:
With 14-Day No-Cook Meal Plan, Recipes and More!

Gretchen Freeman

Table of Contents

Introduction–Keto Diet Handbook

Over the years, excessive weight gain has served as a problem for so many people. While weight gain in itself isn't bad, excessive weight gain has led to the development of extreme medical diseases like cancer and diabetes. To control weight gain and to prevent the continuous development of these diseases, various weight-loss strategies and diet plans have been developed by medical practitioners. Amongst these plans is the reliable Ketogenic Diet.

What is the Keto Diet?

The Keto diet is a high fat and low carbohydrate diet that helps to burn body fat, lose weight, and improve the general health of the body system. The Keto diet supports a drastic reduction of carbohydrate foods and increased addition of fatty foods. This reduction of carbohydrates in the body system puts the body in a metabolic state known as Ketosis.

What is Keto?

Keto allows the body to produce ketones, which serve as an alternative fuel supply for the body when the body experiences a short supply of glucose. High levels of fatty foods and low levels of carbohydrates enhance the production of ketones, which helps the body rely on fat already stored. This process of fat conversion puts the body in the state of Ketosis.

Ketosis

As most body cells prefer to make use of sugar as the main source of energy, the introduction of Keto diet into the body system causes the body to release ketones in the bloodstream, thus giving the body an alternative source of energy. The body's inability to draw energy from sugar that is provided from carbohydrate meals causes a breakdown of fat into ketone bodies, which are now used by the body cells to generate and supply energy to the body through the bloodstreams. This continuous activity is known as Ketosis.

While the body is in the metabolic state of ketosis, the body becomes extremely efficient in fat burn, blood sugar reduction, and insulin levels reduction. Unlike other diet plans, the Keto diet plan gives a satisfying feeling, thus leaving the consumer filled all through the day. While fasting can also cause the body to go into the state of ketosis, it doesn't produce a lasting result as the Keto Diet.

Types of Keto Diet

Different types of Ketogenic diet cause the body to go into a state of Ketosis. While these Keto diet plans have few variations, they all have a common feature of high fat and low carb.

They include:

Standard Ketogenic Diet: The Standard Ketogenic Diet is centered on fatty foods like avocado, meats, fish, olive oil, and butter, low carb foods like melon, non-starchy vegetables, and a moderate amount of protein foods. SKD should contain no set limit of fat, about 40-60g of protein and 20-50g of low carbs food per day. Not only does it promote weight loss, but this diet plan also improves health.

Targeted Keto Diet: Although the targeted Keto diet is quite similar to the standard Keto diet, it is more common amongst athletes who live on the Keto diet but need more sugar. Those who follow this Keto diet plan need more energy when involving the body in active activities, but they burn off the additional carbohydrates during a workout. TKD includes up to 80g of carbohydrates every day.

Cyclical Keto Diet: Cyclical Keto Diet plan is one that involves cyclical incorporation of Keto diet. Those who choose this Keto diet plan cycle in and out of Ketosis. They undergo five days of Ketogenic diet and two days of high-carb diet that includes dairy products, starchy veggies, and whole grains every week. Athletes also use this diet to replenish glucose lost during workout sessions.

High Protein Ketogenic Diet: The HPKD includes a higher amount of protein than the standard Ketogenic diet. Despite an increase in the amount of protein, this diet maintains a higher amount of fatty foods and a very low amount of carbs. Although this modified Keto diet doesn't result in ketosis as protein can also be converted to serve as a source of fuel supply, it still results in weight loss.

Benefits of Keto Diet

It aids in drastic weight loss: Reduction in the intake of carb meals results in the loss of water used in the body system, which results in weight loss. However, continuous placement on the Keto diet results in speedy weight loss because the body now relies on fat rather than sugar. Despite the weight loss, Keto diet doesn't cause hunger due to the inclusion of meals high in protein.

It supplies fuel to the brain and strengthens the brain: Ketones have the ability to supply the brain with 70% of its energy needs. The release of these ketones in the bloodstream provides the brain with immediate fuel that is needed to enable the overall functioning of the body system. An increase in the intake of fatty foods also keeps the brain running effectively. A study released on the effect of Keto diet on the brain states that Keto diet can effectively improve the memory and protect the brain from cognitive decline.

It stabilizes blood sugar level: When carbohydrate is taken, the digestive system converts the carbohydrate to blood sugar—glucose—which is stored and used by the body. Excessive intake of carbohydrates causes the blood sugar to spike, thus resulting in an unstable blood sugar level. However, switching to a Keto diet changes this. Switching from high carb meal to high-fat meal stabilizes the blood sugar level, thus resulting in the lower levels of insulin in the blood, and stabilization of other hormones in women. Diabetics with high blood glucose levels also get to stop taking their medications when they switch to Keto diet.

Keto diet protects the heart and prevents heart disease: For a day meal plan which includes breakfast, lunch, and dinner, the Keto diet contains less or no more than 50g of carbohydrates. This reduction in the number of carbs increases high-density lipoprotein or good cholesterol, thus turning on the anti-inflammatory pathway that protects the heart from heart diseases. This diet also reduces fat molecules in the blood, thus preventing any case of coronary heart disease.

Keto diet reduces inflammation: Inflammation is the body's reaction to a harmful invader. In view of an invasion, ketones produce few free radicals when the anti-inflammatory pathways open. Although inflammation is a natural response, chronic inflammation can cause cancers and heart diseases. To promote this advantage, the Keto diet is usually filled with unprocessed foods, healthy fats, fresh and organic vegetables.

Increased energy levels: Energy level tends to slump when the source of energy is from carb meals. But when the source of energy is fatty foods, the brain never runs out on a constant supply of energy. The metabolic state of ketosis also helps to create a lot of mitochondria (energy factories) in the brain, thus sustaining the cells and organs in the body.

It plays a vital role in disease prevention and treatment: With Keto diet, adults with metabolic syndrome get to treat symptoms like abdominal obesity, high triglycerides, elevated blood pressure, and increased blood sugar levels; people with type 2 diabetes get their blood sugar level stabilized; people with type 2 bipolar disorder get their mood stabilized; obese individuals get to lose belly fat and shed more weight; older adults with dementia get to experience better cognitive and memory functioning, and women with Polycystic Ovary Syndrome (PCOS) get to experience little or no risk of diabetes and obesity.

Keto diet improves body composition: Keto diet doesn't only aid in weight loss, it also aids in the increment of muscle mass due to the consumption of a higher amount of protein. Bodybuilders who aim to build muscle mass go for a targeted ketogenic diet rather than the standard ketogenic diet.

What to Eat on a Keto Diet?

The human body can enter into the metabolic state of ketosis within the first three days of being placed on a Keto diet. This state can lead to a drastic reduction in weight gain as the depletion of glycogen causes the body to drop water weight. Although the complete switch to Keto diet for weight loss is very good for human health, studies have revealed that people find it difficult to maintain a low carb, high-fat diet for more than 12 months. Not only is it difficult to eat with family members, but Keto dieters also find it difficult to go out with friends.

While it has proven difficult for some, those who desire to achieve a healthy milestone that can speedily be achieved through the Keto diet fixate their minds on eating a meal with a high amount of fat, fair amount of protein, and very low amount of carbohydrate.

Low carb:

A Keto meal should only contain at most 10 grams of carbohydrates or 20-50g of carbohydrates in all meals (breakfast, lunch, and dinner) per day. These carbohydrates should be from high fiber, above the ground vegetables, and water-rich fruits, to enhance hydration and to keep the digestive system in continuous operation.

Examples:

Low-carb vegetables: Broccoli, bell pepper, asparagus, avocados, spinach, and mushrooms are vegetables that are extremely low in carbohydrates.

These low-carb vegetables contain a high amount of vitamin C and antioxidants that protect the body against cell-damaging free radicals. Consumption of broccoli and cauliflower has also been associated with the decrease in risk of heart disease and cancer. The low-carb, above-ground vegetables can be fried in olive oil and consumed to replace rice, pasta, potatoes, and other high-carb meals.

Proteins:

To burn calories and to build body mass, it is best to get a minimal amount of protein. Eating less amount of protein can cause the body to turn muscle tissue into fuel, thus lowering the number of calories you burn and the amount of muscle you build. In the same light, the inclusion of a high amount of protein can also put undue stress on the kidney. Cheese, eggs, Greek yogurt, pork, chicken are types of proteins that should be found in a Keto diet meal.

Examples:

Fish and Seafood: Fish is rich in protein, Vitamin B, potassium, and selenium. Fatty fishes like mackerel, tuna, and salmon also contain a high level of fats, which increase omega 3 fats—fats that reduce insulin sensitivity and increase the blood sugar level.

Greek Yogurt: Plain Greek yogurt contains at least 12g of protein. As it is rich in protein and calcium, its intake reduces appetite and promotes fullness.

Meat and Poultry: On the ketogenic meal plan, poultry is a staple. Poultry and fresh meat contain a high amount of vitamin, potassium, selenium and zinc. It is best to include chicken, fish, and beef in any Keto diet as they are organic and healthier than processed meats like meatballs and sausages, which contain up to 5% carbohydrates.

Eggs: Eggs contain a high amount of Vitamin B, protein, antioxidants, and minerals. More so, they contain properties that make consumers have a lower response to ghrelin—the hunger hormone—thus causing them to feel full. They also contain zeaxanthin and lutein—antioxidants that protect the health of the eyes. Egg yolks contain choline—a satisfying nutrient that contains a high amount of fat-burning properties.

Fats: Full fat is the center of every Keto diet meal. The meal composition of a Keto diet should contain up to 165g of fats per day with a focus on the inclusion of unsaturated fats like olive oil, nuts, and flaxseed oil rather than some saturated fats from butter, red meat, and lard.

Cheese: Cheese is a very good fit for a ketogenic diet due to its high-fat content and low-carb content. Cheese also contains conjugated linoleic acid—fat linked to improvement in body composition and steady fat loss. Continuous addition of cheese to the Keto diet plan also helps to strengthen the body and aids in reducing the loss of muscle mass.

Others:

Avocados: Avocados are highly healthy and nutritious. Per serving, they contain about 2g of net carbs and up to 20 minerals and vitamins. Avocados contain a high amount of healthy monounsaturated fatty acids and serve as a source of Vitamins C, E, K, potassium, and magnesium. The fat gotten from avocados informs the brain to turn off appetite, thus keeping the body full and satiated.

Olive oil: Olive oil contains a very high content of oleic acid, which helps to reduce the risk of any heart disease. As it contains no iota of carbs, olive oil is known to be best for salad dressings.

Nuts and seeds: By containing a high amount of fiber, nuts and seeds cause the absorption of fewer calories. Although they are very healthy, nuts and seeds contain a varying amount of carbs.

- An ounce of almonds contains 3g net carbs

- An ounce of Brazil nuts contains 1g net carb

- An ounce of pecans contains 1g net carb

- An ounce of walnuts contains 2gs net carbs

- An ounce of chia seeds contains 1g net carb

- An ounce of flaxseeds contains 1g net carb

- An ounce of sesame seeds contains 3gs net carbs

Berries: Due to the high content of carbs in fruits, fruits are usually avoided in a Keto diet. But, berries are exempted. Unlike other fruits, berries have low carb and high fiber content. Berries also contain antioxidants that reduce inflammation and protect the body against diseases.

- 3.5 oz. of blackberries contain 5gs net carbs

- 3.5 oz. of blueberries contain 12gs net carbs

- 3.5 oz. of raspberries contain 6gs net carbs

- 3.5 oz. of strawberries contain 6gs net carbs.

What to Drink on a Keto Diet

Just as there are things to eat on a Keto diet, there are also things to drink on a Keto diet.

In the beginning stages of the metabolic state of ketosis, the hydration status of the body begins to shift. Aside from exhausting glycogen storage due to the restrictive consumption of carbs, the inability to consume processed foods that are high in sodium also affects the fluid balance of the body. This makes hydration difficult for people on the Keto diet, especially during the early stages. To keep the body hydrated and healthy, there are things to drink during this process.

Here Are the Things to Drink on the Keto Diet

Water: Water should be taken at regular intervals. The body cannot function well when it is dehydrated. More so, muscles find it difficult to make use of nutrients without water. Water can be taken with ice or taken with natural flavorings like lime or cucumber. Salt can also be added when a headache is being experienced.

Tea: Without the addition of sugar or sweetener, tea is carb-free and calorie-free. Tea is also rich in antioxidant flavonoids that promote health. Whether it is black, green, orange, pekoe, herbal, or mint tea, any tea can be taken. However, it is best to take caffeine-free herbal tea during the day.

Bone Broth: Sipping a liquid that contains brewed bones and connective tissues from chicken and fish is a healthy way of maintaining a Keto diet. By simmering the bones in water, nutrients, fat, and other tissues are released in the water. By sipping that water, these nutrients and electrolytes get transferred to the body. A steaming cup of bone broth contains up to 13 calories and about 2.5g of protein. Bone broth is hydrating and satisfying.

Coffee: Coffee without sugar or sweetened milk is excellent for Keto dieters. For Keto dieters who crave the fat supplied by the heavy cream, unsweetened heavy cream should be added to the coffee.

Nut Milk: Cashew milk, almond and coconut milk contain less than a gram of carbohydrate. So, they are safe to drink for Keto dieters.

A Keto diet meal basically contains 5-20g carbs, 20-25% protein and 70-75% fat per day. To maintain the metabolic state of ketosis, it is best for Keto dieters to avoid high carb foods like sugar which can be found in sports drinks, fruit juice, soft drinks, sweets, candies, chocolate bars, doughnuts, frozen treats and packaged goods. Starchy foods (bread, pasta, potatoes, rice, chips, legumes and certain root vegetables), beer and fruits that contain sugar.

Side Effects of Keto Diet

The Keto diet has retained its position as a diet that aids in weight loss, decreased hunger, and reduction in the risks of cancer and other heart-related diseases. However, its switch from the usual metabolic state to the metabolic state of ketosis tends to reveal certain side effects in dieters. While some Keto dieters do not experience any side effects, some do. Essentially, the side effects of Keto diets vary among dieters.

Here are the possible side effects a Keto dieter may experience and how they can be managed/alleviated:

- Keto Flu: Keto flu is common at the early stage of ketosis. Keto dieters may begin to experience weakness, stomach upset/constipation, nausea, and headache due to the fact that their body is beginning to use fat rather than carbohydrates to produce energy. Keto dieters who experience Keto flu should take restrain from strenuous activities till their body adapts to the change. It is also important to change the water and mineral balance of the body by adding a little salt to the water before drinking it in order to make up for the loss of salt. Usually, Keto dieters do not experience the flu after a week of consistent consumption.

- Frequent Urination: As the body system burns through glucose in the first two days of being on a Keto diet, Keto dieters tend to release a lot of water. More so, as the kidney begins to excrete sodium upon the reduction in insulin circulation, Keto dieters may feel the need to urinate more. However, Keto dieters need not worry as the frequent urination stops when the body stops burning through the stored glycogen.

- Dizziness: As the body releases more water when burning through glycogen, the body also tends to release minerals like magnesium, potassium, and sodium. Unavailability of these minerals in the body causes dizziness, fatigue, and light-headedness. However, Keto dieters who do not want to experience it can prevent it by including in their Keto diet foods low in carbs but rich in potassium like broccoli, poultry, fish, avocados and leafy greens. For drinks, leafy greens, coconut milk, blueberries, coconut butter, and avocado can be used to make healthy smoothies.

- Reduction in Blood Sugar Level: Reduction in blood sugar level, which is also known as hypoglycemia, is another side effect that is common to Keto dieters that are previously used to consuming a higher amount of carbohydrate every day. Since the body is used to a high intake of sugar, reduction may lead to hypoglycemia, thus causing the Keto dieter to feel tired or shaky for a while. Just like other side effects, this side effect is temporary and may no longer occur after the first week of being placed on a Keto diet.

- Constipation: Ketosis also affects the way the digestive system functions. As the digestive system tries to adapt, constipation may occur. Constipation can be stopped by an increased intake of foods high in fiber, non-starchy foods, salt, and water.

- Muscle Cramps: Muscle cramps, especially leg cramps, occur when there is a loss of minerals. Keto dieters may also experience frequent cramps in the first week due to the release of minerals. Cramps can be prevented, and mineral loss can be reduced with an intake of more water and salt.

- Smelly Breath: Due to the intake of foods low in carbs, Keto dieters may also experience the smell of acetone (one of the ketone bodies that has a smell similar to a nail polish remover) on their breath. This smelly breath goes away in a few days to two weeks. But in a more extended situation, it is important to:

  o Keep the breath fresh by brushing regularly

  o Drink plenty of water frequently

  o Subside the smell by using a breath freshener

- Heart Palpitations: Keto dieters, especially those with low blood pressure, may experience heart palpitations as a result of the reduction in the fluid circulating in the blood, which is caused by the reduction of salt and water. To put a stop to this, it is best to drink more and more water and add more salt to the food.

- Reduction in Physical Performance: Dehydration, salt and the switch to the metabolic state of ketosis tend to trigger a change in physical performance. As it may be difficult for the body to easily adjust to its new diet, it may take time to perform as required. Keto dieters who experience this side effect are usually athletes. It is best for athletes to try to exercise more while in the transition to enable quick and easy adaptation.

While the side effects of Keto diet vary among dieters, there is no doubt that all the effects can easily be prevented or eliminated by the intake of more water and salt. As these side effects may be inevitable, it is best to tackle them, using natural methods of salt and water intake.

How to Lose Weight on a Keto Diet

The restriction of carbohydrates in meals causes the body to go into the metabolic state of ketosis, where ketones are burnt to supply fuel to the body. At this stage, Keto dieters tend to experience a reduced appetite, thus enabling the consumption of fewer calories, which ultimately results in weight loss. Not only do Keto dieters lose weight based on the consumption of fewer calories, but they also lose weight rapidly, especially in the first week due to the loss of water.

The rate at which Keto dieters lose weight on Keto differs. While weight loss may be obvious in one Keto dieter, it may not be so obvious in another Keto dieter. Usually, shedding of fat and weight loss become more steady and stable after the first week of Keto. However, as the Keto dieter gets close to their weight goal, the rate at which weight loss occurs tends to slow down. This is because Keto dieters tend to review daily calorie intake upon a decrease in weight.

Keto dieters have the ability to sculpt themselves into the shape they desire. However, this can only be done with a well-formulated Keto diet plan, discipline, and consistency.

Here is how to consistently lose weight on a Keto diet:

- Track your calories: Tracking your calories will help you know the effectiveness of the Keto diet. Track your calories using applications like MyFitnessPal to help you see your weight loss/gain progress graph and to help you know whether you are eating the right amount of carbohydrates, protein, and fats every day.

- Have a macronutrient target: You can have a macronutrient target by making use of a Keto calculator. A macronutrient calculator will help you maintain your calorie deficit.

- Fast intermittently: Intermittent fasting is known as a natural supplement for Keto dieters. For intermittent fasting, you can either skip over breakfast or lunch to induce extra time of fasting or incorporate an eating window technique where you fast for a number of hours and eat for a number of hours or totally go into extended fasting periods where you do not eat for 24 – 48 hours. For eating windows, you can schedule 6 hours eating and 18 hours fasting with specificity on eating between a particular time—12pm and 6pm—while you fast all through the remaining hours. Since the body cannot take in more than it should at a particular time, intermittent fasting helps to limit the calorie intake.

- Do not cheat on your Ketogenic diet: Cheating on your Keto diet by consuming a high carb for just a day will cause a rapid weight gain. If you crave sugar, you can indulge in Keto snacks.

- Avoid eating foods you are allergic to. If you are sensitive to certain foods, avoid including them in your Keto meal. Eating such foods can affect your health and weight loss progress.

- Look out for hidden carbs: Some low carb foods may actually contain hidden carbs. While you think you have been consuming a low-carb food, you may have been consuming a high carb meal. So, ensure you check the carbs from meats, butter, and vegetable before consuming them.

- Eat the right amount of protein: Overeating protein can lead to a decrease in ketone levels, and an increase in insulin levels while eating less protein can lead to burning muscle rather than fat. In your Keto meal, protein should be more than carbs but less than fat.

- Take MCTs (Medium Chain Triglycerides): MCTs are types of saturated fats that can be converted to ketones. They serve as supplements. They increase the level of satisfaction, reduce the amount of food intake, enhance cognitive performance, and boost energy levels.

- Consume more of high-fat dairy: High-fat dairy contains a high amount of conjugated linoleic acid, which is known to improve fat loss. High-fat dairy can be gotten from dairy, beef, and grass-fed cows.

14-Day No-Cook Meal Plan

14-Day No-Cook Meal Plan—10-Minute Preparation Time

When you are on a Keto diet, you can either cook your meals or opt for easy Keto meals that don't require you to go through the cooking process. No-cook Keto meal plan is suitable for people who do not have enough time to cook, and those who want to avoid cooking separate meals in their homes.

Week 1

Monday

Breakfast	Lunch	Dinner
Bacon, egg salad with tomato dressing	Chicken salad stirred in olive oil and cheese	Smoked salmon with steamed broccoli stirred in butter

Tuesday

Breakfast	Lunch	Dinner
Cheese rollups	Avocado, bacon and goat cheese salad	Chicken with basil boats

Wednesday

Breakfast	Lunch	Dinner
Keto milkshake	Grilled beef and cheese plate	Seafood salad with avocados

Thursday

Breakfast	Lunch	Dinner
Sugar-free yogurt with peanut butter, cocoa powder, and stevia	Cooked beef in coconut oil and vegetables	Chicken with cream cheese, pesto, and vegetables

Friday

Breakfast	Lunch	Dinner
Eggs with mayonnaise	Caesar salad	Keto cheeseburger

Saturday

Breakfast	Lunch	Dinner
Bacon and eggs	Cheese rollups with vegetables	Spicy Italian salad

Sunday

Breakfast	Lunch	Dinner
Coffee	Tuna salad with boiled eggs	Burger patties with creamy tomato sauce

Week 2

Monday

Breakfast	Lunch	Dinner
Egg with avocado, salsa, pepper, onion, and spices	Antipasto salad	Turkey, avocado, and lettuce stirred in cream cheese and olive oil

Tuesday

Breakfast	Lunch	Dinner
Scrambled eggs	Shrimp and broccoli	Keto salami and brie cheese plate

Wednesday

Breakfast	Lunch	Dinner
Unsweetened latte	Smoked salmon plate	Tortilla with ground beef and salsa

Thursday

Breakfast	Lunch	Dinner
Egg muffins	Shrimp, eggs, spinach, and tomatoes with olive oil, salt, and pepper	Pork chops with green beans and garlic butter

Friday

Breakfast	Lunch	Dinner
Avocado, eggs, and bacon	Salad in a jar	Crabmeat and egg plate

Saturday

Breakfast	Lunch	Dinner
Tuna salad with capers	Chicken wings with creamy broccoli	Salmon filled avocados

Sunday

Breakfast	Lunch	Dinner
Keto bread with eggs	Fish with baked beets	Chicken wings with cheese dressing

33 Keto Recipes

1. Turkey with cream cheese sauce

- 1½ lbs. turkey breast

- 2 tbsps. butter

- 7 oz. cream cheese

- 2 cups heavy whipping cream

- ⅓ cup small capers

- 1 tbsp. tamari soy sauce, salt, and pepper

➢ <u>Instruction</u>

o Preheat the oven to 350F.

o Season the turkey.

o In a large oven-proof frying pan, melt half the butter and fry the turkey all round.

o Place the turkey in the oven to cook well. Afterward, place it on a plate.

o In a small saucepan, pour turkey drippings, add whipping cream and cream cheese, then stir and boil for a while.

o Reduce the heat, and let it simmer till it thickens. Add salt, pepper and soy sauce.

o In another frying pan, heat the remaining butter and cook the capers until crispy.

o Serve butter-fried turkey with sauce and fried capers.

2. Pimiento cheese meatballs

- ⅓ cup mayonnaise

- 1 ½ lbs. ground beef

- 1 egg

- 1 tbsp. butter

- Salt and pepper

- 1 tsp. chili powder, or to taste

- ¼ cup pimientos

- 1 tbsp. Dijon mustard

- 1 pinch cayenne pepper

- 3 oz. grated cheddar cheese

➢ Instructions

o In a large bowl, mix all ingredients except beef, egg, pepper, salt, and butter.

o Add egg and beef to the mixture in the bowl.

o Add salt and pepper to taste.

o Form meatballs and fry in oil.

o Serve with mayonnaise or green salad.

3. Baked salmon with pesto

Sauce

- 1 cup mayonnaise
- 4 tbsps. green pesto
- ½ cup full-fat Greek yogurt
- Pepper and salt

Salmon

- 4 tbsps. green pesto
- 2 lbs. salmon
- Pepper and salt

➢ Instructions

o Grease the baking dish.

o Place salmon on it, skin side down.

o Rub pesto, salt, and pepper.

o Bake in a pre-heated oven at 400° F for 30 minutes.

o Stir the sauce ingredient in another bowl.

o Serve sauce with salmon.

4. Pork roast with creamy gravy

- 1 ½ cups heavy whipping cream
- 2 lbs. pork roast
- 1 bay leaf
- 2 ½ cups of water
- 5 black peppercorns
- ½ tsp. salt
- 2 tsps. dried thyme
- 2 garlic cloves
- 2 tbsps. olive oil
- ½ tsp. black pepper
- 1½ tsps. ginger
- 1 tbsp. paprika powder

➤ Instructions

o In a deep baking dish, place the pork, and add salt, water, bay leaf, thyme, and peppercorns. Cover with foil and leave in the preheated oven for 7–8 hours.

o Afterward, separate the pork from the juice.

o From 210° F, increase the oven heat to 430° F.

o In another bowl, grate garlic and ginger, add pepper, herbs, paprika powder, and oil and stir well.

o   Rub the pork with the mixture.

o   Place the pork in a baking dish and leave in the oven till it is golden brown—10–15 minutes.

o   For the gravy, strain the pork juice to remove solids.

o   Boil for a while.

o   Add whipping cream and boil. Then reduce the heat to simmer for 15–20 minutes.

o   Serve pork roast with creamy gravy.

5. Oven-baked chicken in garlic butter

- 3 lbs. whole chicken
- ½ tsp. ground black pepper
- 2 tsps. sea salt
- 2 garlic cloves, minced
- 6 oz. butter

➢ Instructions

- Preheat oven to 400° F.
- Season the whole chicken with salt and pepper, inside-out.
- Place the chicken on a baking dish.
- Over medium heat, melt butter and garlic.
- Drizzle the garlic butter over the chicken inside-out.
- Sprinkle with garlic butter every 20 minutes.
- Bake for 1-1:30 minutes.
- Serve with any side dish.

6. Shrimp salad with hot bacon

- 2 oz. chopped bacon

- 6 oz. fresh spinach

- 2 chopped boiled eggs

- 1 lb. peeled shrimp

- 1 tbsp. butter

- **Bacon dressing**

- ½ cup bacon fat or olive oil

- ¼ cup apple cider vinegar

- ½ tbsp. Dijon mustard

- Salt

- Ground black pepper

➢ Instruction

o Wash spinach, dry the leaves and divide between plates.

o Fry chopped bacon on high heat.

o Divide bacon and egg in spinach filled plates.

o Remove moisture from shrimp. Melt butter in a pan, add shrimp and cook for 5 minutes.

o Divide shrimp among the plates and sprinkle cheese.

o In another saucepan, heat the bacon fat, and sprinkle the vinegar and other ingredients.

o Pour the hot bacon fat over the salad plates.

7. Tuna salad with capers

- 4 oz. tuna in olive oil

- Finely chopped ½ leek

- ½ tsp. chili flakes

- Salt and pepper

- ½ cup of mayonnaise

- 2 tbsps. crème fraiche

➢ Instructions

o Drain tuna of olive oil.

o Mix tuna with all ingredients.

o Serve with boiled egg or sesame crispbread.

8. Fresh spinach frittata

- 5 oz. diced bacon

- 8 oz. fresh spinach

- 8 eggs

- ½ cup heavy whipping cream

- 2 tbsps. butter

- 5 oz. shredded cheese

- Salt and pepper

➢ Instructions

o Preheat oven to 350° F and grease baking dish.

o Fry bacon in butter. Add spinach and stir.

o Set bacon aside. Whisk egg and cream and pour in a baking dish.

o On the egg and cream mixture, add bacon, spinach, and cheese. Add salt and pepper.

o Bake until it is golden brown.

o Serve with any side dish.

9. Cheesy omelette

- 6 eggs
- 2 tbsps. heavy whipping cream
- 3 oz. shredded cheese
- 2 oz. butter
- 5 oz. diced, smoked deli ham
- ½ yellow onion, finely chopped
- ½ green bell pepper, finely chopped
- Salt and pepper

➤ Instruction

o Whisk egg and heavy cream together.

o Add salt, pepper, and shredded cheese and mix together.

o In a large frying pan, melt butter. Then, add diced deli ham, onions, and pepper and cook together.

o Add egg mixture and fry until omelet is a little firm.

o Reduce the heat, sprinkle the remaining cheese, fold the omelet and gently place on a dish.

o Serve with a green salad.

10. Scrambled eggs

- 2 eggs
- 1 oz. butter
- Salt and pepper

➤ Instruction

o In a bowl, mix the egg with salt and pepper.

o Melt butter in a frying pan over medium heat.

o Add the eggs and stir till they are cooked.

11. Keto banana waffles

- 1 ripe banana
- 4 eggs
- ¾ cup almond flour
- ¾ cup of coconut milk
- 1 tbsp. ground psyllium husk powder
- 1 pinch of salt
- 1 tsp. baking powder
- ½ tsp. vanilla extract
- 1 tsp. ground cinnamon
- Coconut oil or butter

➢ Instruction

o In a bowl, mix all ingredients together.

o Make the waffles using a waffle maker or fry in a pan.

o Serve with berries or hazelnut spread.

12. Keto bread

- 1¼ cups almond flour

- 2 tsps. baking powder

- 3 egg whites

- 5 tbsps. ground psyllium husk powder

- 1 tsp. sea salt

- 1 tsp. cider vinegar

- 1 cup of water

➢ Instructions

o Preheat the oven to 350°° F.

o In a large bowl, mix all the dry ingredients.

o Boil water.

o Add vinegar and egg whites to the dry ingredients and mix well.

o Using a hand mixer, add boiling water and mix.

o Add little at a time to avoid softening the dough.

o Rub hands with oil, cut dough into sizes, then roll and place each on the baking sheet.

o Depending on the size of the dough, bake for 50-60 minutes.

13. Keto muffins

- 2 eggs
- 2 tbsps. coconut flour
- ½ tsp. baking powder
- 3 tbsps. butter or coconut
- A pinch of salt

➤ Instructions

o Mix coconut flour, baking powder and a pinch of salt.

o Add the eggs and mix until it is well combined.

o In frying, add the butter to melt.

o Scoop in about 3 dollops of the batter.

o Fry for some time and turn to fry the other side.

o Serve with a milkshake and your favorite toppings.

14. Cauliflower rice 5g

- 1½ lbs. cauliflower
- 3 oz. butter or coconut oil
- ½ tsp. turmeric (optional)
- ½ tsp. salt

➢ Instructions

- Shred the cauliflower head, using a grater.
- Melt butter or use coconut oil, add the cauliflower and cook for about 10 minutes.
- Add salt and turmeric (optional).
- Serve with low carb veggies.

15. Butter fried green cabbage

- 1½ lbs. shredded green cabbage
- 3 oz. unsalted butter
- Salt and pepper

➢ Instructions

- Using a sharp knife or a food processor, shred the cabbage into bits.
- Melt butter in a large skillet over a medium heat.
- Add cabbage and stir-cook until the cabbage edges become golden brown.
- Reduce the heat, then add pepper and salt to taste.

16. Broccoli Mash

- 1½ lbs. broccoli
- 4 tbsps. finely chopped fresh basil or parsley
- 3 oz. butter
- 1 garlic clove
- Salt and pepper

➤ Instructions

o Chop, peel and cut broccoli into pieces.

o In lightly salted water, boil broccoli for a few minutes.

o Drain the water.

o In a food processor, blend broccoli with other ingredients.

o Add salt and pepper to taste.

o Add more oil and butter as desired.

o Serve hot.

17. Coconut salmon with napa cabbage

- 1¼ lbs. salmon
- ½ cup unsweetened shredded coconut
- 1 tsp. turmeric
- 1 tsp. kosher or ground sea salt
- ½ tsp. onion powder
- 4 tbsps. olive oil
- 1¼ lbs. napa cabbage
- 4 oz. butter
- Salt and pepper
- Lemon (as desired)

➢ Instruction

o In a bowl, mix unsweetened shredded coconut, turmeric, onion powder, and salt.

o Cut the salmon into pieces and toss into the coconut mixture bowl.

o On medium heat, fry coated salmon in melted butter until it is golden brown.

o In another pan, fry wedged cabbage lightly in olive oil. Then add pepper and salt.

o Melt the remaining butter and drizzle on the coated salmon and cabbage while serving.

18. Chicken Tonnato

Tonnato sauce

- 2 tbsps. small capers
- 4 oz. tuna in olive oil
- 2 garlic cloves
- ¼ cup chopped fresh basil
- 2 tsp. dried parsley
- 1 tbsp. lemon juice
- ½ cup mayonnaise
- ¼ cup olive oil
- ½ tsp. salt
- ¼ tsp. ground black pepper

Chicken

- 1½ lbs. chicken breasts
- Water
- Salt
- 7 oz. leafy greens

➢ Instructions

o In a blender or food processor, mix all the tonnato sauce—capers, tuna, garlic cloves, chopped fresh basil, dried parsley, mayonnaise, lemon juice, olive oil, salt, and black pepper.

- In a pot, add salt to the chicken breast and boil till the chicken is cooked. Place the chicken on the cutting table for about 10 minutes.

- Place the leafy greens on the plate, the sliced chicken on it and drizzle in sauce.

- Serve with lemon or capers.

19. Keto baked eggs

- 3 oz. cooked ground beef
- 2 eggs
- 2 oz. shredded cheese

➢ Instructions

o Preheat oven to 390° F.

o Arrange beef in a baking dish.

o Make a hole in the middle of the grounded beef.

o Crack in eggs and sprinkle shredded cheese.

o Bake for 10-15 minutes.

o Serve when it is cool.

20. Goulash Soup

- 1 yellow onion
- 3 garlic cloves
- 8 oz. celery root
- 1 red bell pepper
- 1 lb. ground lamb or ground beef
- 1½ oz. butter or 3 tbsps. olive oil
- 1 tbsp. paprika powder
- ¼ tsp. cayenne pepper
- 1 tbsp. dried oregano
- ½ tbsp. crushed caraway seeds
- 1 tsp. salt
- ¼ tsp. ground black pepper
- 14 oz. crushed tomatoes
- 2½ - 3 cups of water
- 1½ tsps. red wine vinegar

➢ Instructions

o Finely peel and chop vegetables.

o On medium heat, sauté onion and garlic with plenty of oil or butter.

o Add the meat and allow to cook thoroughly.

o Add other ingredients except for the red wine vinegar. Stir and pour 2 cups of water. Allow it to cook.

o Reduce the heat and allow it to simmer for 10 minutes.

o Add vinegar and the remaining water.

o Serve with mayonnaise or sour cream.

21. Butter burgers

- 1 lb. 80/20 ground beef
- 1 tsp. salt
- ½ tsp. ground black pepper
- ¼ red onion
- 1 fresh jalapeño
- 1 tomato
- 1 avocado
- 1 butter lettuce
- 1 oz. cheddar cheese (2 slices per burger)
- 1½ oz. sliced butter

➢ Instructions

- On medium heat, pre-heat the grill for 20 minutes.
- In a separate bowl, mix beef, pepper, and salt together.
- Chop onions and jalapeno into smaller pieces. (To avoid extra spice, remove the jalapeno seeds.)
- Add onions and jalapeno to the beef and mix with your hand.
- Form two hamburger patties.
- Grill on both sides for 5-7 minutes.
- Thinly slice tomatoes. Spoon out the flesh.
- When all is ready, place burger on 3-4 lettuce leaves, and then sprinkle slices of cheese and butter, a slice of avocado and tomatoes, salt and pepper.
- Wrap and serve.

22. Chicken fritters

- 1 cup coconut oil or avocado oil, for frying

- 1 small yellow onion, diced

- 2 celery stalks

- 1 tsp. salt

- 1 tsp. dried oregano

- 1 tsp. ground cumin

- 13 oz. skinless, boneless chicken thighs

- 2 large eggs

- ¾ cup fine coconut flour

➤ Instructions

o Over a medium heat, heat oil in a large skillet.

o In a food processor, add onions, celery stalk, and spices. Mince well.

o Add chicken thighs and eggs.

o Process till it forms a thick paste.

o Pour coconut flour in a plate.

o Scoop the paste on coconut flour and mold till it forms a ball.

o Repeat the same process till the paste is used up.

o Gently add fritters in the oil and fry till each side is golden brown.

o Remove with a slotted spoon and place on a paper towel to remove oil.

o Serve with sauce.

23. Cheese dressing

- 5 oz. blue cheese
- ¾ cup Greek yogurt
- ½ cup mayonnaise
- ½ cup heavy whipping cream
- Salt and pepper
- 2 tbsps. finely chopped fresh parsley

➢ **Instructions**

- Place cheese in a bowl and divide into chunks.
- Add heavy whipping cream, yogurt, and mayonnaise. Mix well.
- Allow it to sit for a while.
- Add salt and pepper. Add parsley and mix well.
- Try the dressing on cheeseburgers, salad, or avocados.

24. Spicy chorizo with creamy green cabbage

Creamed green cabbage

- 1½ lbs. green cabbage
- 2 oz. butter
- 1½ cups heavy whipping cream
- Salt and pepper
- ½ cup finely chopped fresh parsley
- ½ tbsp. lemon zest

Fried Chorizo

- 1½ lbs. chorizo
- 2 tbsps. butter, for frying

➢ Instructions

o Over medium heat, fry chorizo in butter.

o Using a knife or food processor, shred cabbage.

o Remove chorizo and keep warm.

o Cook cabbage with the remaining butter. Stir intermittently until the cabbage is golden brown.

o Add whipping cream. Reduce the heat and allow it to simmer till the cream reduces.

o Sprinkle salt and pepper to taste.

o Add parsley and lemon zest.

o Serve with fried chorizo.

25. Avocado bacon and goat cheese salad

- 8 oz. goat cheese
- 8 oz. bacon
- 2 avocados
- 4 oz. arugula lettuce
- 4 oz. walnuts

Dressing

- 2 tbsps. lemon juice
- ½ cup mayonnaise
- ½ cup olive oil
- 2 tbsps. heavy whipping cream
- Salt and pepper

➢ Instructions

o Place baking paper in baking dish and place in the oven to preheat.

o Slice the goat cheese, place in the baking dish and bake until it is golden brown.

o Fry bacon until it is crispy.

o Cut avocado into pieces, and place it on top of the arugula lettuce. Then add fried bacon, and goat cheese and sprinkle nuts.

o In a blender, mix the dressing together. Add pepper and salt to taste.

26. Frozen yogurt popsicle

- 8 oz. frozen mango, diced

- 8 oz. frozen strawberries

- 1 cup full-fat Greek yogurt

- ½ cup heavy whipping cream

- ½ tsp. vanilla extract

➢ Instructions

o Leave the strawberries and mango to soften for 15 minutes.

o In a blender, mix all ingredients.

o Serve immediately as soft ice cream or harden using an ice cream maker or pour into popsicle molds and freeze for hours.

27. Blueberry smoothie

- 14 oz. canned, unsweetened coconut milk
- 3 oz. frozen blueberries or fresh blueberries
- ½ tbsp. lemon juice
- ½ tsp. vanilla extract

➤ Instructions

o Mix all ingredients in a blender till the paste is smooth.

o Serve chilled.

28. Coleslaw

- ½ lb. green cabbage

- ½ lemon, the juice

- ½ tsp. salt

- ½ cup mayonnaise or vegan mayonnaise

- pinch of fennel seeds (optional)

- 1 pinch pepper

- 1 tbsp. Dijon mustard

➤ Instructions

o Shred the cabbage using a cheese slicer.

o Pour in a bowl and add lemon juice and salt.

o Stir and allow to sit for 10 minutes.

o Drain excess juice.

o Mix cabbage, mayonnaise and Dijon mustard (optionally).

o Add seasoning to taste before serving.

29. Chicken coconut

- 2 tbsps. coconut oil
- ⅓ lb. broccoli
- 1 yellow onion
- 1 lb. cooked chicken breasts or turkey
- 14 oz. coconut milk or coconut cream
- 1½ tbsps. green curry paste
- 1 tbsp. peanut butter
- Salt and pepper
- 1½ oz. salted peanuts, for topping

➢ Instructions

o Peel and thinly cut onions.

o Peel the stem of broccoli and cut broccoli into thin rods.

o Pour plenty of oil in sauté pan. Stir-fry broccoli and onions for a few minutes.

o Add salt and pepper to taste.

o Slice chicken meat and add to the pan.

o Add coconut milk, curry paste, and peanut butter and stir.

o Sprinkle a little salt and pepper.

o Add peanuts and serve hot or warm.

30. Coconut porridge

- 1 egg
- 1 tbsp. coconut flour
- pinch of ground psyllium husk powder
- pinch of salt
- 1 oz. butter or coconut oil
- 4 tbsps. coconut cream

➤ Instructions

o In a medium-size bowl, add coconut flour, psyllium husk powder, egg, and salt.

o Melt butter and coconut cream over low heat.

o Whisk egg mixture and combine with melted butter and cream.

o Having achieved thick texture, serve with coconut milk or cream.

31. Chia pudding

- ½ tsp. vanilla extract
- 1 cup unsweetened canned milk or almond milk
- 4 tbsps. chia seeds

➢ <u>Instructions</u>

- o In a jar, add all ingredients and blend.
- o Cover the jar and place it in the fridge for up to 4 hours.
- o Ensure the pudding thickens.
- o Serve with cream, milk or berries.

32. Granola

- 2½ oz. unsweetened shredded coconuts
- ½ cup almond flour
- 8 oz. almonds
- 4 tbsps. sesame seeds
- 4 tbsps. coconut oil
- 4 tbsps. pumpkin seeds
- ¼ cup sunflower seeds
- ¾ cup flaxseed
- ½ tbsp. turmeric
- 1 tbsp. ground cinnamon
- 2 tsps. vanilla extract
- 1 cup water

➢ Instructions

o With a sharp knife, chop nuts and mix together with other ingredients in a bowl.

o Pre-heat the oven to 300° F.

o On a baking sheet, spread the mixture and roast in the oven for 15-20 minutes.

o Remove from the oven and stir.

o Return to the oven for another 15-20 minutes.

o When the granola feels dry, remove and allow to cool.

o Serve with Greek Yoghurt.

33. Keto turkey plate

- 1 sliced avocado
- 2 oz. lettuce
- 3 oz. cream cheese
- 6 oz. turkey
- 4 tbsps. olive oil
- Salt and pepper

➢ Instructions

o Place avocado, lettuce, cooked turkey and cream cheese on a plate.

o Drizzle olive oil and season to taste with salt and pepper.

Food Shopping and Pantry List for Keto Dieters

Adhering to a specific diet makes shopping difficult because you would have to shop for specific things. As a Keto dieter, things get much more difficult because you have to strictly search for items low in carb and high in fat.

To make shopping fun and easier for you, here are some of the things you should include on your list:

Meats

- Pork
- Chicken
- Bacon
- Seafood
- Turkey
- Beef
- Ham
- Ground beef

Dairy

- Butter (grass-fed)
- Hard cheese
- Heavy cream

- Greek yogurt

- Mayonnaise

- Sour cream

- Cottage cheese

- Soft cheese

Eggs

Flour

- Almond flour

- Coconut flour

- Psyllium husk

Fats

- Coconut oil

- Olive oil

- Avocado oil

- MCT oil

- Bacon fat

- Ghee

- Cocoa butter

- Lard

Vegetables

- Broccoli

- Asparagus

- Cauliflower

- Cabbage

- Garlic

- Pumpkin

- Onion

- Pepper

- Ginger

- Spinach

- Tomatoes

- Mushrooms

- Lettuce

- Zucchini

- Artichokes

- Radishes

- Okra

Nuts and seeds

- Almonds

- Pecans

- Flaxseeds

- Walnuts

- Pumpkin seeds

- Chia seeds

- Sunflower seeds

Fruits
- Avocados
- Lime

- Lemon

- Berries

- Unsweetened coconut

Unsweetened nut butters

- Peanut butter

- Almond butter

- Macadamia nut butter

- Almond butter

Pantry list

- Chicken broth

- Herbs and spices

- Pork rinds

- Low carb salad dressings

- Bone broth

- Coconut aminos

- Baking cocoa powder

- Parchment paper

- 100% unsweetened chocolates

- Pink Himalayan sea salt

- Baking powder

- Baking Soda

- Apple extract

- Vanilla extract

- Swerve Confectioners

- Swerve Granular sweetener

- Almond extract

- Caramel extract

- Lemon extract

- Maple extract

- Vanilla stevia

- Egg white protein powder

- Swerve brown sugar

- Xanthan gum

- Cream of tartar

Unsweetened shredded coconut

Action Plan and Tips for Keto Dieters

Action Plan

- Set goals for your weight loss: Goals should include a timeframe.

- Set measurable standards: This should include checking your weight at least once in two days.

- Set actionable steps: Actionable steps should include clearing out your kitchen and re-filling it with Keto foods.

- Set a budget: Eating on a budget will help you achieve your Keto dream without spending a lot of money.

- Set dates you would go on intermittent fasting.

- Incorporate the Keto meal calendar to help you consume the right amount of carbs, protein, and oil.

Tips for Keto Dieters

- Always use low-carb, high-fat ingredients to make meals.

- Avoid stressful exercises but exercise frequently.

- Drink a lot of water.

- Try intermittent fasting.

- Reduce the stress in your life—avoid exhausting activities.

- Maintain a proper sleep schedule.

- Eat more salt to avoid electrolyte imbalance.

- Regularly supplement with MCT oil.

- Try ketones supplement like exogenous ketones.

- Measure your carb intake.

- Measure your ketones to know if you are in ketosis.

- Clear out your kitchen. Replace the items cleared with Keto foods.

- Maintain the amount of protein you consume.

Conclusion

Different types of diet plans surely exist, but there is no diet plan that gives the result a Keto diet can give. Not only does a Keto diet aid in weight loss, but it also helps to improve certain conditions like cognitive decline and type 2 diabetes.

A Keto diet should include a high amount of healthy fat, a moderate amount of protein, and a very low amount of carbohydrates for the body to go into the metabolic state of ketosis.

Some people experience side effects, and some do not. However, those who experience side effects get better in days. Depending on your level of consistency, the Keto diet result begins to show in no time.

Although going on a Keto diet isn't easy, carefully following all the information in this handbook will help you achieve your goals.

Made in the USA
Coppell, TX
03 December 2024

41726842R00042